Positive heart remodeling

Positive heart remodeling

Dr Jerzy George Dyczynski

dyczynskitelehealth.co

I dedicate this book to my patients and cardiology teachers equally.
I am full of gratitude for their contribution to the growth of my knowledge about the heart and holist c Cardiology.

CONTENTS

Introduction

And I will give you a new heart, and I will put a new spirit in you. I will take out your stony, stubborn heart and give you a tender, responsive heart. Ezekiel 36, Verse 26-27.

How often do you focus your thoughts on your heart, trying to feel and communicate with it? Perhaps your interest in your heart has been sparked by chest pain, shortness of breath, or heart palpitations. If so, now is the perfect time to realize that your heart is your best friend and needs more appreciation. By reading this text, you have already started the process of transforming your heart and initiating its positive remodeling.

Let us take a closer look at your heart, your best companion, and what it does for you every day. Your heart is an incredible organ that works harmoniously with your brain and body. Its connection to your family and social network is indispensable for your physical health. It beats approximately 40 million times a year, creating a powerful magnetic field within and around your body. As your body's powerhouse, the heart provides energy equivalent to powering a strong light bulb at its peak performance.

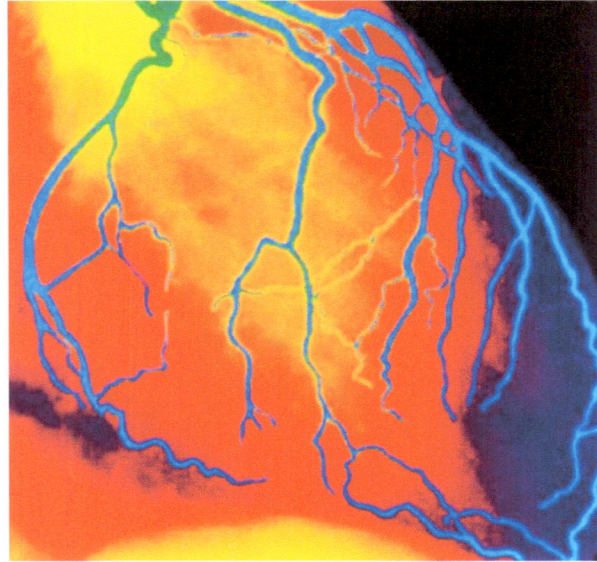

**Picture 1. The coronary arteries displayed using
Magnetic Resonance Imaging MRI.**

Your heart generates about 3 kilograms of renewable energy every 24 hours and has the remarkable ability to heal and regenerate itself through the production and release of stem cells, even while you sleep. Embrace the idea that your heart is intelligent and allow this awareness to grow. Imagine that your intelligent heart can clear blockages, resolve coronary artery spasms, and normalize an irregular heartbeat. With cooperation, your heart can even spontaneously stop your heart palpitations. Like a best friend, it requires the right circumstances and a healthy environment to function optimally. When your heart struggles to meet the demands of modern life, it can change in size and shape, becoming enlarged and more rigid. These changes are known as adverse heart remodeling, and they can adversely affect your entire body. Symptoms of this condition may include swelling in the legs, shortness of breath, chest discomfort, and low energy levels. If you experience chest pressure, palpitations, or pain in your arm, shoulder, or lower jaw, your heart is trying to send you a message. This chest pain, known as "angina pectoris," translates to "a feeling of constriction in the chest" in Latin. If left untreated, it can cause damage to the heart muscle and potentially lead to a heart attack.

Adverse remodeling is increasingly common, affecting more than 600 million people worldwide, and you could be among them. If you are seeking an effective and practical solution, you've come to the right place, and your transformation can begin here and now. A 21st-century, evidence-based, holistic health model is available to help you direct your intelligent heart toward reversing adverse remodeling.

Adverse remodeling often results from prolonged stress related to work or family, insufficient physical activity, and the constraints of modern life. These factors can lead to shallow breathing, poor oxygenation, and fatigue. If not addressed, they may cause heart palpitations, chest discomfort, and pain in the arms and hands. It is vital to you to recognize these signs and not ignore or misinterpret them. Awareness and timely action can enable you to manage your heart health and prevent or halt the progression of adverse heart remodeling.

Hormonal imbalances and high levels of stress can also lead to irregular heartbeats and spasms in the coronary artery, signaling early signs of heart issues. If you leave these symptoms unaddressed, they can contribute to a decline in your heart's precision and flexibility, worsening adverse remodeling.

Additionally, external factors such as global warming, climate change, and modern lifestyles, which expose you to environmental toxins, microplastics in water, and unpredictable weather, can trigger abnormal heartbeats or coronary artery spasms—key contributors to adverse heart remodeling.

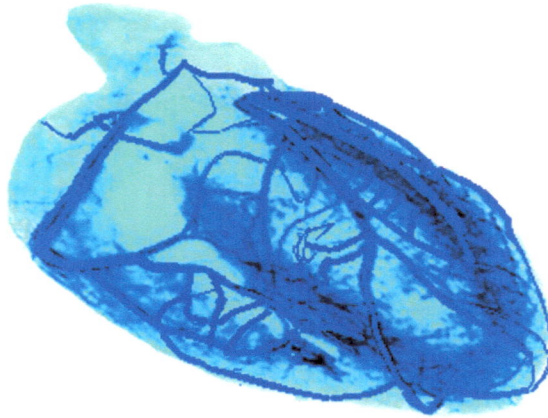

**Picture 2. Heart with displayed rich coronary vessels
network supplying the muscle of the left chamber.**

It is less known that the adverse remodeling of your heart can also affect the brain, causing it to become dormant and less active. An inactive, dormant brain can impact your thinking and memory, leading to confusion or even a mini stroke. In this abnormal situation, the heart cannot pump enough blood to the brain.

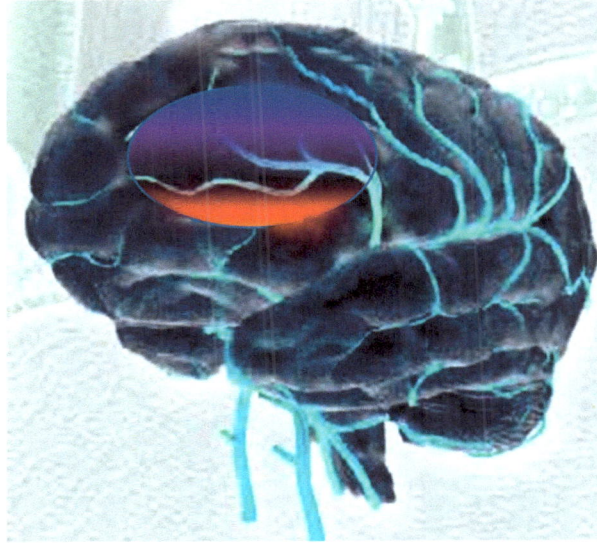

Picture 3. Dormant brain.

The greatness of the new information age extends beyond scientific research. It is personal. Your access to up-to-date global cardio knowledge is making it easier for you to make informed decisions about your heart health. Healthcare knowledge is no longer exclusive to medical professionals. You no longer need to rely solely on practitioners for treatment plans and information that may be influenced by their personal and professional views. Today, it is important for you to take charge of your heart and your cardiovascular health.

While healthcare professionals are essential to a successful healthcare system, your personal engagement and expanding knowledge will give you more control over your heart health. This new level of confidence as a knowledgeable observer of your body and your healthcare environment will allow you to take charge and help design your individual treatment program.

Regarding cardiovascular health, no one better understands your heart's impressive power to combat infirmity and to maintain your perfect health than you.

Western medicine has always taught us that our bodies are mainly unchangeable and primarily fixed in form. Besides noticeable changes like weight gain, loss or changes in strength and flexibility, it has been widely accepted that our organs do not change apart from age-related deterioration.

Only recently have scientists discovered the brain's plasticity. It can perfectly recover from trauma or infirmity and change its functionality according to your body's demands. Your heart has an extraordinary ability to adapt, transform, and renew itself, even surpassing the brain's plasticity. Your mission is to support your self-organizing system of your heart and body. Your goal is to unlock your heart's intelligence, which embodies its inherent wisdom and adaptability. By doing this, you can reassess your heart health and prioritize your intelligent heart in your new lifestyle.

Holistic medicine and medical physics have uncovered several facets of your heart's intelligence that have the power to reverse adverse remodeling. Incorporating these facets has the potential to bring about profound positive changes in your heart's functionality. These changes will work together to counteract adverse heart remodeling, instilling in you hope and fostering renewed optimism.

2

Knowledge of your heart

He has made everything beautiful in its time. He has also set eternity in the human heart: yet no one can fathom what God has done from the beginning to the end. Ecclesiastes Chapter 3, Verse 11.

In a metaphysical sense, knowledge of the heart refers to God's understanding of man's heart and the special knowledge that people have deep within their hearts.

While we typically think of the heart as a pump for circulating blood, it actually serves other vital functions as well. The best example is the production of five types of hormones in your heart. They can overwrite any other hormones release in your body. It is a part of supremacy of the heart in the functionality of your body.

Recent breakthroughs in cardiology, quantum physics, and medical physics have confirmed the heart's crucial role in the human body, including its connection to spirituality and memory. Memory, a sophisticated human function, significantly shapes one's personality. In a pivotal year 2000 performed study, the authors revealed a connection between the heart and human memory. The study found that the personality and consciousness of a heart donor went to the personality of the recipient. This was a pivotal moment in our understanding of the heart's intelligence.

Recipients of transplanted hearts could recall the specific life circumstances of the donors despite never having had any contact with them. This study represented a significant advancement in recognizing the heart as an organ capable of inheriting memories.

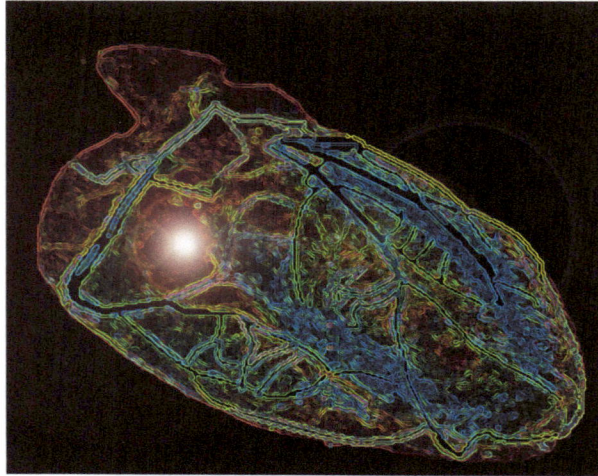

Picture 4. Metaphysical heart. Artistic vision.

These ground breaking findings validate traditional spiritual beliefs and establish a profound connection between spirituality and modern cardiology. This alignment of modern cardiology with traditional medical beliefs in natural healing offers a sense of unity in medicine.

The broad impact of modern communication and information technology will largely determine the course of humanity in general and, more specifically, what will happen to each of us individually and, quite specifically, to you and me. Healing your intelligent heart and reversing its adverse, negative remodeling is personal.

As medical science advances at a rapid pace, you find yourself in an information age that is shaping your destiny. You are not just a patient but a key player at the forefront of the changing landscape of modern heart science. Understanding the intelligence of your heart has the power to transform your healing and your active role in it.

Your intelligent heart has the capacity to reverse its negative, adverse remodeling, which is great news for you. Your transformation will take a few months. It requires a treatment plan, an understanding of your heart's physical and spiritual aspects, and, most importantly, your commitment to start today.

Cutting-edge medical knowledge offers you the promise of holistic heart health. One of the most significant benefits of the information age is your ability to access the healing power through expanded knowledge about your intelligent heart and your self-organizing body. The "hibernating myocardium" is one of the most recent discoveries in scientific research and one of the underlying conditions leading to your heart's adverse remodeling.

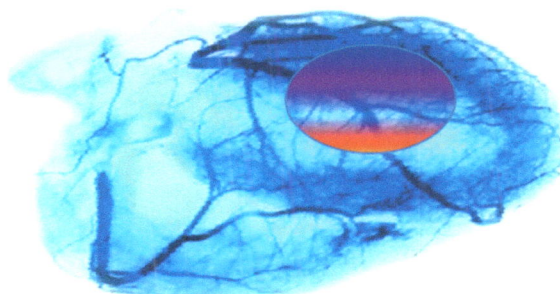

Picture 5. Hibernating myocardium.

Hibernating myocardium is functional and refers to a part of your heart muscle. This region of the heart muscle became less responsive to nerve signals due to a lack of oxygen and a slowed metabolism. The hibernating area has lower activity, resembling a state of sleepiness or laziness. The cause of the hibernation is mainly related to a spasm of the coronary artery. In the next chapter, let us look more closely at the mechanism of the spasms in the coronary arteries before we proceed to the hibernating myocardium.

3

Spasms of coronary arteries

My heart grew hot within me; as I mused, a fire burned. I spoke with my tongue. Psalm 39, Verse 3.

It is essential for you to realize that your coronary vessel producing the spasm is only narrowed and not blocked. Coronary artery spasms are mostly linked to active, hot plaque, a build-up of fats, cholesterol, debris, fragments of proteins, dead cells and other stuff in the artery walls.

Approximately half of the global population has plaques with cholesterol deposits in their arteries, and even children can have plaques. Men and women around their 40s are prone to significant plaque build-up and to the development of their vulnerability. A spasm in a coronary artery with a vulnerable plaque will typically cause the hibernating myocardium, a vegetative state of the part of your heart.

The spastic Angina pectoris is known also as a variant or Prinzmetal Angina pectoris, coined after the name of the doctor, who discovered and described it. Generally speaking, people experiencing spasms of the coronary artery have fewer risk factors for coronary artery disease.

Coronary artery spasms happen when the small muscles that control blood flow in the coronary arteries do not produce enough Nitric Oxide (NO) and do not get enough oxygen. Nitric oxide relaxes the muscles in the blood vessels of the heart and is an important signaling molecule in the body. It is produced from essential amino acids found in your food and oxygen from your breathing.

Nitric oxide, a common air pollutant found in car exhaust fumes, has been discovered to have remarkable benefits for the body. It protects your heart, stimulates your brain, and can kill bacteria.

Despite its short 10-second lifespan, nitric oxide's unique nature as a signal molecule made it subject to extensive research. Contemporary research has revealed that it plays a fundamental role in the cardiovascular system, a fact that is often overlooked.

Nitric oxide also regulates blood pressure, and its presence is crucial in preventing Angina pectoris and stopping the formation of blood clots. Furthermore, it is vital for brain function and linked to memory.

Additionally, NO is a key player in your body's defense system. It aids in fighting infections, becoming toxic to invading bacteria and parasites when produced by your white blood immune cells. This incredible molecule is also utilized by blood cells to defend the body against tumors, making its role in your body truly indispensable.

A spasm in your coronary artery can be triggered by various factors, including insufficient or shallow breathing and emotional stress. Other potential triggers include increased plaque temperature due to inflammation, toxic influences, and mineral imbalances, especially between Magnesium and Potassium. Additionally, an intense stress reaction with adrenaline over-stimulation can also lead to a spasm of an artery in your heart.

Spasms develop in extreme weather, with volatile temperatures , including hot or cold, intense emotional stress, and stimulating substances like caffeine, alcohol, drugs, certain medications, high cholesterol, and high consumption of energy drinks or cocaine.

A plaque in a coronary artery can become vulnerable, hot and reactive if viruses or bacteria inflame it. The vulnerable plaque and its hot reactivity can cause spasms, further narrowing, and reduced blood flow.

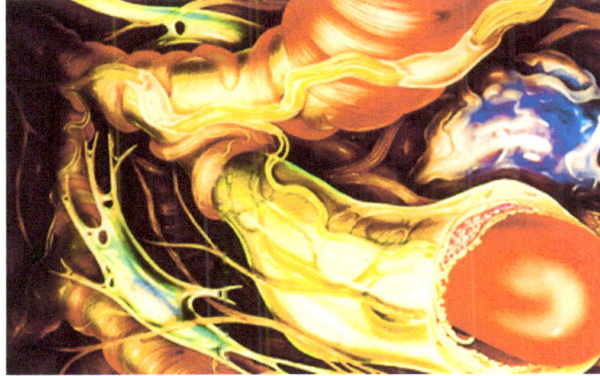

Picture 6. A spasm of a small coronary vessel.

The image above shows a small blood vessel within the coronary artery system. This coronary vessel is constricted due to spastic muscle activity, which reduces blood flow. A single red blood cell is visible in the center of the vessel. In addition to the blood vessels, connective tissues are present, including a fibroblast located in the bottom left corner. Fibroblasts are essential cells that help form connective tissue. Above the constricted vessel, there is an active immune blood cell. Another blood vessel, which is functioning normally, can also be seen, surrounded by a specialized type of muscle known as vasculature.

Your heart has two big coronary arteries: the left and right. The third significant coronary artery is between them. It supplies blood to your left lower chamber known as ventricle and your left upper chamber known as atrium. Numerous smaller branches originate from the big coronary arteries and an unaccountable number of tiny coronary vessels exist in your heart's micro-circulation. Each coronary artery has its own, tiny regulating muscle known as vasculature to regulate the amount of blood flow.

The symptom of coronary artery spasms is chest pain, which may feel for you like burning, fullness, or pressure in your chest, along with heart palpitations. The pain may also spread to your arms, neck, jaw, shoulder, or back. It is important for you to know that even a coronary artery spasm in a small coronary artery can produce intense chest pain.

Your understanding of the role of plaque in your actions related to your heart health is fundamental. The presence of plaque in the heart does not always lead to symptoms of Angina pectoris or a heart attack. However, when the plaque becomes vulnerable, hot, and active, it can cause spasms. If a spasm lasts longer unchecked, it can produce a blockage and potentially damage your heart. This underscores the absolute importance for you to be aware and cautious about the functional spasms of coronary arteries. They carry a potential risk to the integrity of your intelligent heart.

Diagram of discomfort caused by coronary artery disease. Pressure, fullness, squeezing, or pain in the center of the chest. Discomfort can also be felt in the neck, jaw, shoulders, back, or arms, as depicted below.

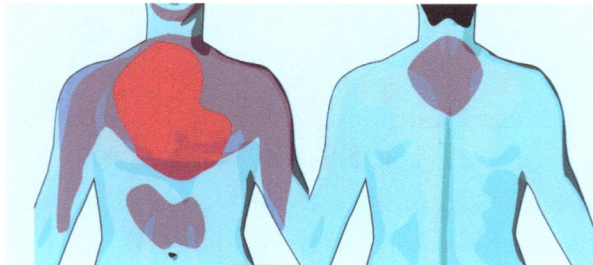

Picture 7. By Ian Furstin Wikipedia.

Unlike Angina pectoris, which results from a blockage of a coronary artery and is characterized by a suffocating sensation in the chest in a resting position or during physical activity, coronary artery spasms occur unexpectedly, often at rest, even in pleasant outer circumstances. Chest pain from a coronary artery spasm occurs mainly at night or early morning when your breathing is weaker.

The use of Nitroglycerin spray by people with angina pectoris is a globally accepted practice. Nitroglycerin has a fascinating history. Mr Alfred Nobel, a figure of great historical significance, developed its use as a blasting explosive by mixing it with an absorbent, particularly 'Kieselgur,' a form of silica from the soil. He named this explosive dynamite and patented it in 1867. From his amassed fortune, he funded the Nobel Prize Foundation. Alfred Nobel suffered from a heart condition marked by paroxysms of intense chest pain known as Angina pectoris, and his doctor prescribed him Nitroglycerin. This medication would later prove to be a life-saving treatment for many heart conditions.

Nitroglycerin converts in your body to Nitric Oxide, abbreviated NO. The small molecule NO causes rapidly the smooth muscle within your coronary blood vessel to relax and to release the spasms. It is a powerful medicine that acts as a signalling molecule in your body.

NO was proclaimed as the Molecule of the Year by a prestigious scientific journal Science in 1992 and then the research about NO as a signalling molecule in the cardiovascular system was awarded with Nobel Prize in Medicine in 1998.

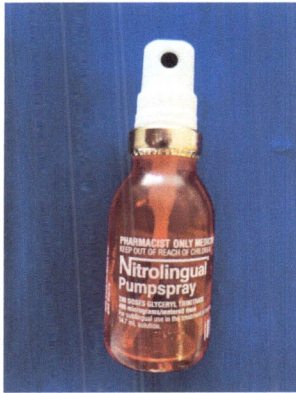

Picture 8. Nitroglycerin spray.

Nitroglycerin spray is a valuable resource for your management of the chest pain during episodes of Angina pectoris, a condition caused by narrowed or spasming coronary vessels that supply blood to your heart.

There is a worldwide agreement about the use of Nitroglycerin in Angina pectoris. It is reflected in the recommendations about its application through patients in numerous national cardiac societies, including the European Society of Cardiology, the American College of Cardiology, the American Heart Association, the American College of Physicians, the American Association for Thoracic Surgery, Preventive Cardiovascular Nurses Foundation of Australia & Cardiac Society of

Australia and New Zealand, and the Asian Pacific Society of Cardiology, which represents 23 cardiology societies in the Asia-Pacific region. The Indian Heart Association and the Chinese Society for Cardiology also support this practice.

Nitroglycerin is not only a treatment for chest pain but also a tool that you can apply just before daily activities. This can encourage you to take control and prevent episodes of Angina pectoris.

Some patients have found that spraying their chest alleviates angina pectoris and relieves their heart palpitations. This method helps them avoid the sudden decrease in blood pressure that can occur when taking it orally.

4

Hibernating myocardium

Wake up, my heart! Wake up, O lyre and harp! I will wake the dawn with my song. Psalm 57, Verse 8.

Hibernating myocardium is often a result of a spasm in your coronary artery. It refers to a part of the heart muscle that has slowed down the work of contractions. This region of the heart becomes less responsive to nerve signals due to a lack of oxygen and has a sluggish metabolism. The hibernating area has no strength to tense the heart muscle and contract properly. It resembles a state of sleepiness or laziness. Simply put, this part of the heart muscle is essentially *vegetating* to protect itself from heart attack because it does not receive enough oxygen.

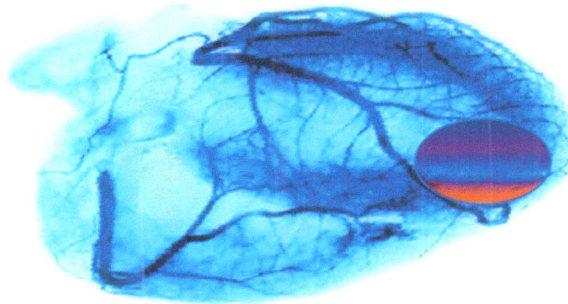

Picture 9. Hibernating myocardium.

Hibernating myocardium is a common and widespread experience that occurs in various forms multiple times over a lifetime of majority of people. Usually, only a small portion of your heart muscles *fall asleep* to reduce the workload and protect your heart from damage. If your heart could not enter the state of hibernation to protect itself, a heart attack would be imminent. Is it not remarkable that your heart has a clever self-protecting mechanism? It remains vital even when waiting for a fresh supply of oxygenated blood to resume normal function. However, if hibernation in your heart is left unchecked, it can last for months or even years. If it lasts longer, it contributes to adverse, negative remodeling.

Vulnerable plaque

He heals the broken hearted and binds up their wounds. Psalm 147, Verse 3.

Atheromatous plaque, also known simply as plaque, is an abnormal build-up in the inner layer of the coronary artery wall that requires focused attention. It is akin to a small wound in the lining of a coronary artery that attracts various substances, essentially acting as a magnet for "stuff." This stuff includes dead cells, debris, cholesterol and other lipids, calcium, and varying amounts of scar tissue, amounting to a swelling in the artery wall. This can encroach into the artery's opening, leading to narrowing and eventually restricting blood flow.

Plaque is a root cause of coronary artery narrowing. Even minimal narrowing of the coronary vessel can trigger spasms that manifest as Angina pectoris.

Picture below shows a microscopic view of the buildup of a plaque in the upper right. The first image in the upper left corner is a small coronary vessel. The upper right corner displays the alarming situation where the plaque is formed and starts to restrict blood flow. In the two images below, an artist's translation in red/orange colors of the actual situation in the micro-circulation captured through a microscope in blue, vividly highlights the stagnation of blood flow caused by plaque building, a concerning health risk.

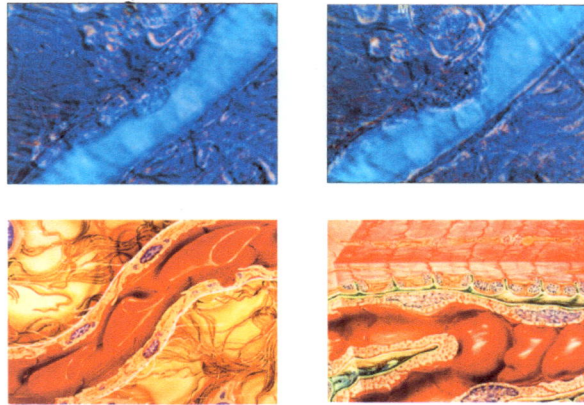

Picture 10. The plaque building up in blue. Artist's vision in red/orange color.

It is important for you to remember that plaque becomes vulnerable when it is infected by bugs or viruses. This infection causes the plaque to become inflamed, making it reactive, prone to spasms, and sometimes rapidly growing. The plaque is only covered by a thin layer separating it from the bloodstream, and if this thin cover tears, it's called plaque rupture. This repeated process of plaque tearing and healing is a factor in developing a solid coronary artery blockage, which can eventually lead to the common appearance of Angina pectoris.

Another factor contributing to plaque vulnerability is slow clot formation. Research on 'vulnerable plaque' shows that these plaques typically have a thin cap over a large fat core and exhibit an inflammatory response.

Your understanding of plaque formation and the immediate recognition of the first signs of plaque vulnerability help you calm and cool down the inflamed plaque. Knowing that the plaque needs more oxygen and calming the inflammation, you can take inspired actions such as practicing more intense breathing, consuming more turmeric-seasoned food, or taking Statin medication. These actions can help relieve chest pain or prevent an approaching episode of Angina pectoris.

Calcium score

For this people's heart has grown callous, they hardly hear with their ears, and they have closed their eyes. Otherwise they might see with their eyes, hear with their ears, understand with their hearts, and turn, and I would heal them. Matthew 13, Verse 15.

Your understanding that plaque is not just a deposit, but an injury in the lining of your blood vessel caused by deposits of cholesterol, eventually inflammation, and sharp Calcium crystals, brings you to the level of 21st-century medical science. Detecting your vulnerable plaque is a task that doctors and specialists are well-equipped to handle. Their expertise and knowledge are mind-blowing. The accumulation of Calcium in the plaque, known as micro-calcification, is a process that can be examined and monitored. An ordinary plaque starts with about 5% Calcium, which can make up to 30% of the healed plaque.

Why does the calcium content in the body increase? This is an important question. The body has a specific method for healing hot, infected, and vulnerable plaques. It cools down the soft, vulnerable plaque and transforms it into a solid mass, securely attached to the artery wall through calcium deposition. The soft, inflamed plaque, which contains various elements such as bacteria, debris, and fat fragments, acts like a magnet, attracting more of these components. Additionally, this plaque can be a source of blood clots or may become torn due to high blood pressure. When this occurs, the bloodstream can carry tiny pieces of the plaque further down the coronary artery, potentially leading to blockages.

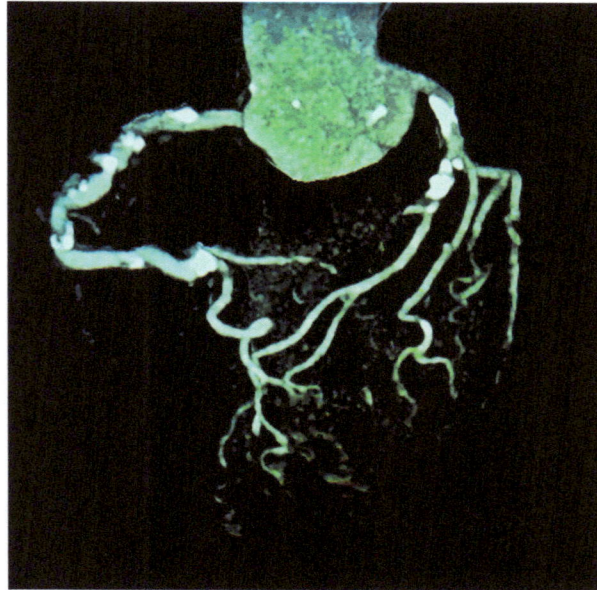

Picture 11. Three dimensional, non-invasive visualization of the CT coronary angiography with Calcium spots.

The modern CT heart scan is a powerful tool that can visualize the coronary arteries, detect the calcium deposits in your coronary artery, and provide a three-dimensional picture of your coronary arteries. This advanced technology helps you with a comprehensive understanding of your cardiovascular health.

A computerized tomography (CT) of the heart, also known as a coronary Calcium score, is a non-invasive method for assessing the deposits of Calcium in the coronary arteries plaques. This specialized CT scan provides heart images for doctors to detect and measure the Calcium content of the plaques in your coronary arteries.

Table 1. Interpretation of coronary calcium score[3]		
Calcium score	Interpretation	Risk of myocardial infarction/stroke at 10 years
0	Very low risk	<1%
1–100	Low risk	<10%
101–400	Moderate risk	10–20%
101–400 and >75th percentile	Moderately high risk	15–20%
>400	High risk	>20%

Picture 12. Agatston score.

The test results you receive from your radiological facility is a score in Agatston units. Dr Arthur Agatston, an American cardiologist and celebrity, developed this method of calculation the Calcium in the coronary arteries. According to the Australian Journal of General Practice, the test helps to assess the risk of heart attack or stroke.

7

Elly's case study

A happy heart is good medicine and a joyful mind causes healing, But a broken spirit dries up the bones. Proverbs Chapter 17, Verse 22.

A plaque is usually filled with 'stuff, a complex mixture of fats, cholesterol, calcium, debris of dead cells, and other substances. The Calcium content in a slightly narrowed coronary vessel plaque is only about 5%. This soft, fatty, and unclean plaque can become a breeding ground for bacteria or viruses, especially when your immune system is compromised. It is important to underline that a weakened immune system can lead to plaque contamination, making it hot, reactive, and vulnerable.

Let us consider Elly's situation, which was about six years ago. She used to lead an unhealthy lifestyle and then experienced her first episode of Angina pectoris with anxiety and palpitations. After visiting her GP, she was referred to undergo a CT calcium score, and upon receiving the report, she visited her referring doctor. Her GP informed Elly that she was at high risk of having a heart attack or stroke.

This news shocked Elly but motivated her to choose a healthy lifestyle. According to the Agatston, Elly's Calcium score was 496, which indicates a higher risk.

Elly started eating healthy food and avoiding alcohol. She also commenced respiratory muscle training, pranayama yoga classes, and acupuncture treatments to lower her stress levels. She also started respiratory muscle training (RMT) using an oxygen concentrator. Elly is proud to have spent over 1,000 hours on RMT training in this way.

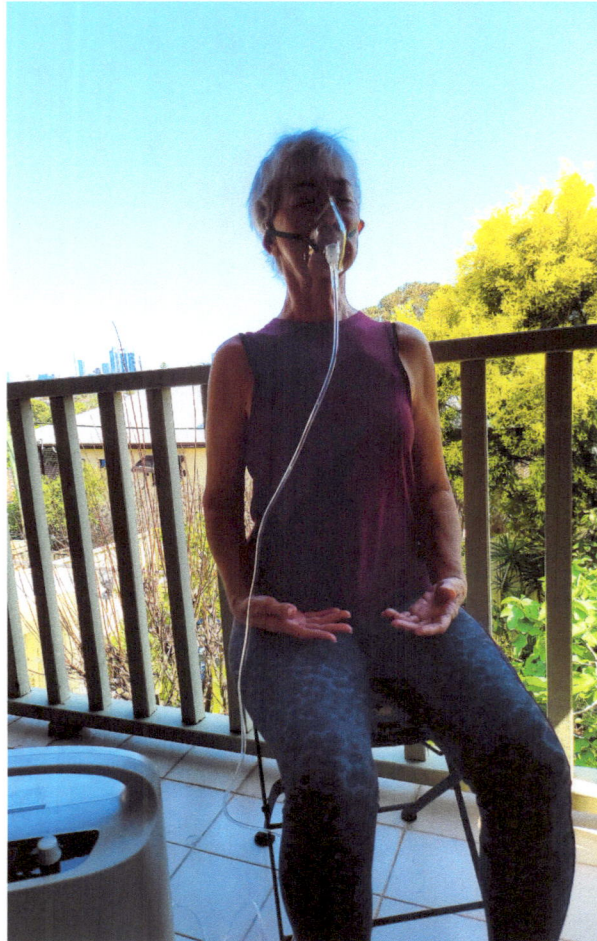

Picture 13. Elly performs her respiratory muscle training.

She has made significant personal and spiritual progress and has maintained her holistic lifestyle for more than six years. Recently, Elly decided to check if her new lifestyle had impacted her Calcium score. She underwent a noninvasive CT angiography heart scan, including the Calcium score.

A CT coronary angiogram examines the arteries supplying blood to the heart. This noninvasive test can reveal vulnerable plaques in the heart's arteries as well as cooled down and calmed calcified plaques. It has been available for about a decade, and about 50 million of these sophisticated CT heart scan screenings have been performed globally in a year. The noninvasive CT heart scan showed a few narrowing of the coronary arteries and an increase in calcified spots. The calculated Calcium score increased to 902. However, the visualized flow in the coronary arteries was sufficient and good.

After the Calcium score increased, Elly visited a specialist Cardiologist. The Cardiologist advised Elly to urgently consider being admitted to the hospital for further diagnostics and eventually for bypass surgery.

This news came as a real shock to Elly given her strong belief that her positive lifestyle changes would improve her health. She decided to undergo a noninvasive diagnostic test on a treadmill with stress echocardiography to assess her heart's vitality and performance under a high load of exercises and visualize her beating heart.

During the test, the technician and cardiologist monitored Elly's performance closely. Despite the increasing workload, Elly experienced no chest pain or shortness of breath. At the peak of her performance, the cardiologist intervened and ran out from her office room, which was separated from the testing room through a big window, and asked Elly:

Do you have any chest pain or shortness of breath?

No, only some muscle pain in my legs and butt replied Elly.

Then the Cardiologist advised the technician to stop the test, as Elly had already reached the predicted load. After the test, the cardiologist informed Elly that there were no issues with the movement of her heart walls and no exercise-induced shortage of blood supply. All this indicated a low risk of developing angina pectoris or a heart attack.

After facing initial challenges, the stress echo test greatly relieved. Elly was reassured and could return home feeling at peace. Elly actively maintains a healthy lifestyle, including a balanced diet, respiratory muscle training, yoga classes, and medical acupuncture treatments.

The Elly's case study suggests that an increase in the Calcium score scan should be considered an indicator of efficient healing of the coronary arteries' vulnerable plaques. Under favorable circumstances, plaque can be healed through increased calcification, making it cold and stable and not putting you at risk of a heart attack.

8

MRI of vulnerable plaque

I the LORD search the heart and examine the mind, to reward each person according to their conduct, according to what their deeds deserve. Jeremiah Chapter 17, Verse 10 .

High-resolution magnetic resonance imaging (MRI) is the leading method for learning more about coronary artery plaques. MRI is highly effective in visualizing and evaluating soft tissues, while CT scans excel at identifying plaque calcification and its extent.

MRI can accurately identify high-risk plaque features such as internal bleeding, chemical composition, lipid concentration, water content, grade of inflammation, and particle movements affected by plaque temperature.

But wait a minute. How can your body be looked through, even to the heart, by applying an external magnetic field?

An MRI scanner interacts with small, naturally occurring mini-magnets in your body's water. These mini-magnets are positively charged hydrogen atoms at the atomic level. Hydrogen, the universe's simplest and most abundant element, comprises 75% of all matter. Your body predominantly consists of water and hydrogen atoms in organic molecules such as fat, sugars, and proteins. Water (H2O), the major component of your body, constitutes 70% of the body's mass. Your body hydrogen protons are a positively charged and spin constantly, generating an electrical charge and a magnetic field.

For instance, it's mind-boggling to comprehend that 1 milliliter of water contains over 6 quintillion protons, which is represented by the number 6,000,000,000,000,000,000,000.

This multitude of mini magnets within your body all have random, chaotic orientations of their poles. Poles of the hydrogen-positive charged protons are the regions at their ends where the magnetic field is most potent.

The phenomenon of the strong external magnetic field penetrating your body and creating order feels impressive. Your body responds positively to the order. It is fascinating and a bonus to have excellent images of your plaques.

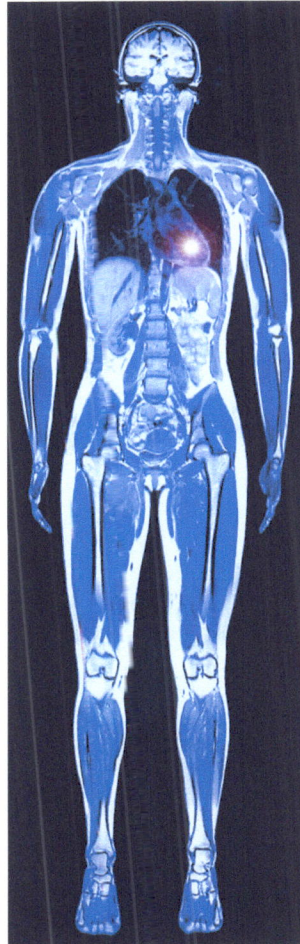

Picture 15. MRI of the full body.

9

Noninvasive CT Cardio scar

God, examine me and know my heart; test me and know my anxious thoughts. See if there is any bad thing in me. Psalm 139, Verse 23.

A non-invasive CT coronary angiogram is a type of heart scan that uses a powerful X-ray machine to take pictures of your heart and the blood vessels that supply it. These images can show if there are any blockages in these blood vessels. The test can also tell if these blockages are made of soft or hard material. It can discern between the vulnerable and calcified plaques. This test is often used to calculate the Calcium score, which can help predict your risk of heart disease.

If you decide to get a referral from your GP and undergo this examination, your heart will be scanned at a high speed to diagnose coronary artery disease. The collected images allow physicians to assess the extent of the plaques in your coronary arteries. Non-invasive CT coronary angiography is usually also used to determine the coronary CT Calcium score.

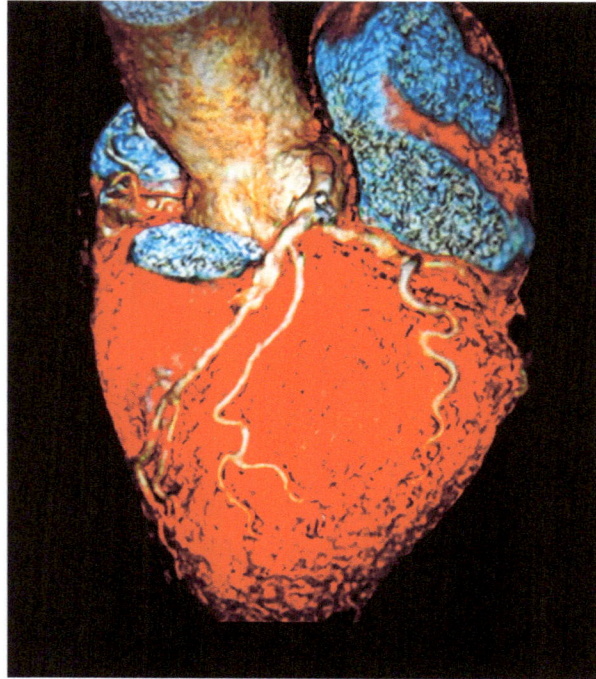

Picture 14. CT coronary angiography.

Are you concerned about radiation? It's a common concern, but during a non-invasive CT coronary angiography, you receive only half the dosage you would with an invasive catheter angiography. These are the only two diagnostic methods available to diagnose plaques and potential blockages in the coronary arteries. The picture above is an example of the detailed heart image generated by the CT coronary angiography, a safe and effective procedure.

10

Blood tests

The blood is God's sign bearing special significance. The blood signified a life had been given and sacrificed. Leviticus Chapter17, Verse 1i.

There are many helpful tests to detect vulnerable plaques and the hibernating myocardium. The most straightforward test is the C-reactive protein CRP in your blood. CRP is a protein produced by the liver. This remarkable organ plays an important role in the body's inflammatory response. The level of CRP rises parallel to the level of inflammation in your body. A high-sensitivity C-reactive protein hs-CRP test is more sensitive than a standard C-reactive protein test. The high-sensitivity test can detect smaller amounts of C-reactive protein in your blood than a standard CRP test. The hs-CRP test can help you assess the risk of developing vulnerable plaques.

You can request the Erythrocyte Sedimentation Rate ESR from your GP. This blood test involves taking a blood sample from you and putting it in a chemical tube to prevent blood clots. The tube is left to stand upright, allowing the red blood cells to gradually fall to the bottom of the tube while the clear liquid plasma remains at the top. The ESR measures the rate at which the red blood cells separate from the liquid plasma and fall to the bottom of the test tube in millimeters per hour. If specific inflammatory proteins cover the red cells, they may stick to each other, causing them to fall more quickly. Therefore, a high ESR indicates the presence of inflammation in your body.

Leukocytes, or white blood cells, are the key defenders of the immune system. They originate from your bone marrow and defend the body against infections and disease. This function should reassure you about your immune system's capabilities. When vulnerable plaques develop more inflammation through contamination by bugs or viruses, the leukocytes enter the plaque to combat the inflammation. An excess of white blood cells in your blood, in the context of coronary artery disease, usually indicates the presence of hot and reactive vulnerable plaques.

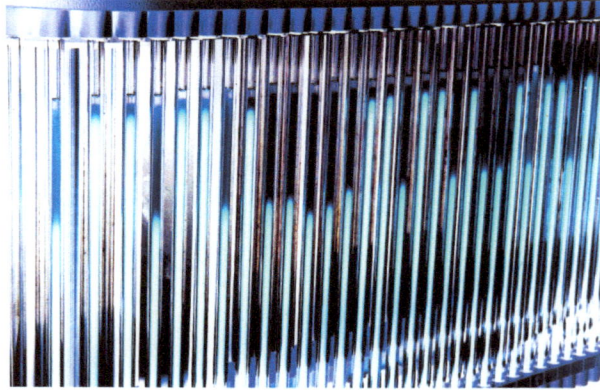

Picture 16. Erythrocyte Sedimentation Rate, ESR Test.
Reverse color view. By MechESR Wikipedia.

Recent research has unveiled the remarkable adaptability of platelets, which can contribute to the development of vulnerable plaques. While the platelets role in your blood is in clot formation and wound healing, they exhibit a wide range of functions, from immunity to cell communication. When a minor injury occurs in the wall of your coronary artery platelets swiftly gather at the site to form a clot.

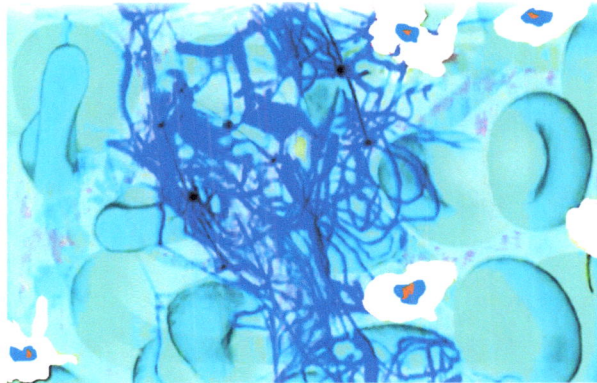

Picture 17. Platelets and fibrin net in a plaque. Reverse color view.

Platelets attract a clotting substance called fibrin to form a net. The clot within a vulnerable plaque is made up of platelets stacked in this net. Platelet levels can be assessed through a full blood count test, which requires a GP referral. If more vulnerable plaques are activated, the circulating platelets in your blood can increase.

A troponin test measures another protein released when the heart muscle is damaged. Studies have shown that elevated troponin levels are common after strenuous exercise in healthy individuals and in other cardiac conditions.

Brain Natriuretic Peptide BNP helps the body to compensate for heart weakness and can indicate the presence of hibernating myocardium. BNP is one of the powerful hormones produced by your intelligent heart. Heart weakness occurs when the heart becomes too weak or stiff due to hibernating myocardium or a scar in the heart wall, preventing it from pumping normally. The most common causes for increased blood BNP are plaques due to coronary artery disease and high blood pressure. A result greater than 100 in one milliliter is abnormal.

11

Cool down your vulnerable plaques

*H*e heals the brokenhearted and binds up their wounds." Psalm 147, Verse 3.

When it comes to cooling down and calming vulnerable plaques, there are two medical approaches to consider: natural and conventional. Combining both can lead to quick and efficient improvement.

Opting for a natural medicine approach to cool down and to calm vulnerable plaques is rooted in increasing your knowledge about your heart health and in boosting your body's oxygen levels.

Your body is a self-organizing system that needs a sufficient amount of oxygen for proper functionality. Recognizing this and delivering more oxygen to your cells puts you more in control of your health. Improving your body's oxygenation and supplying fresh blood with oxygen to the coronary arteries and vulnerable plaques are very important for your heart health.

To ensure this, the best way is to start abdominal breathing in a lying position. This technique will also open the constricted blood vessels in your brain. This can sometimes make you feel light-headed. Therefore, the lying position is the best way to start your respiratory muscle training. You can enhance your oxygen levels through diaphragmatic, abdominal breathing.

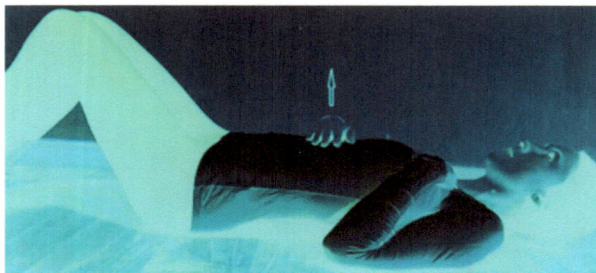

Picture 18. Abdominal, orbital breathing in a lying position. Courtesy of Brittany Giadresco, Nee Ford.

Remember to focus on your breathing during respiratory muscle training. With each inhale, visualize the flow of energy moving up from your crotch through your spine, up to your head, and down to the area between your nose and upper lip. When you exhale, the energy flows from your bottom lip down backe Ford. to your crotch. These two energy channels form the microcosmic orbit. Your lips, mouth, and tongue connect these two energy channels to complete the microcosmic orbit.

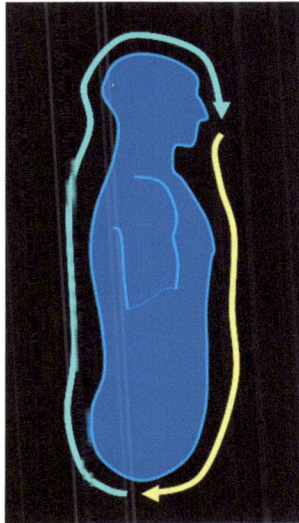

**P.cture 19. Microcosmic
orbit by Bostjan46.
Wikipedia.**

Embrace lifestyle modifications that are not only beneficial but also comfortable and easy to incorporate into your daily routine. These include consuming healthy foods with anti-inflammatory properties, like turmeric, ginger and galangal rots. Experiment with intermittent fasting, and stress-relieving techniques such as: energy channel training, spine flow moves, Pranayama yoga, active meditation or Pilates. The most beneficial relaxation exercises have to focus on abdominal or orbital breathing.

Additionally you can use an oxygen concentrator to increase the oxygen content of the air you breathe during your daily respiratory muscle training RMT.

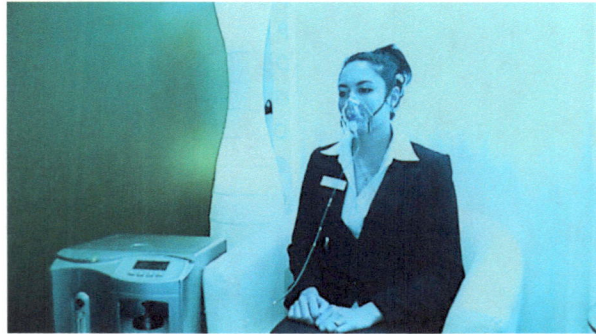

Picture 20. Respiratory muscle training using an oxygen concentrator.

Rest assured, the conventional medical approach to cooling down the plaque to prevent the build-up of the clot and the progress of inflammation is a safe and effective option. It includes the use of lipid-modifying agents like Statins, Nitroglycerin, and Aspirin, which prevent your vulnerable plaque from clot build-up, and blood pressure medications, all of which have been rigorously tested and proven to be beneficial, providing you with a secure and confident treatment plan.

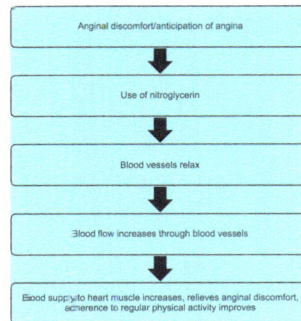

Picture 21. Mechanism of action of Nitroglycerin. Managing Your Angina Symptoms with Nitroglycerin. Courtesy Rainer Hambrecht, MD, FESC Kathy Berra, MSN, ANP; Karen J. Calfas, PhD.

Statins are well-established for treating vulnerable plaques. Statins are originated from a natural source, yeast. Statin therapy straddles the line between natural and conventional medical approaches and can be taken in tablet form or in its natural state. Monascus purpureus is a reddish-purple strain of yeast that produces statins and is used commercially in various industries.

Red yeast rice extract (RYRE) is obtained from the fermentation of a type of yeast found in rice and is marketed as a supplement. It contains an ingredient called monacolin K, which may lower 'bad' cholesterol and is already an ingredient in a statin called lovastatin.

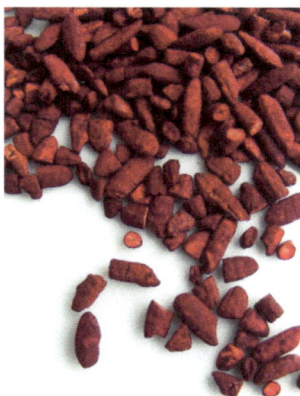

**Picture 22. Red yeast rice
by Fotoos VanRobin.
Wikipedia.**

Well documented studies have shown that Statins treatment can reduce the dimensions of coronary artery plaques, a phenomenon known as plaque regression. This reduction leads to improved clinical benefits, including reduced chest pain, indicating a beneficial effect on stabilizing plaques and demonstrating their effectiveness in calming and stabilizing vulnerable plaques. Plaque stabilization is a significant outcome of this treatment, making the plaque less likely to tear and cause a bleeding. This effect is likely due to a reduction in the plaque's lipid-rich core, decreased inflammation, and accelerated calcification with reduced platelet reactivity.

Lipid-modifying agents like Statins have a comprehensive pleiotropic effect, meaning they have more than one positive effect beyond just lowering cholesterol. This leads to a wide range of health benefits for you. Statins improve cellular respiration, enhance plaque stability, reduce inflammation, and prevent clot formation. These additional effects of Statins help you to calm and stabilize the plaques, providing significant personal benefits by easing symptoms and relieving chest pain, leading to less frequent occurrences of Angina pectoris.

In terms of additional medication, Calcium antagonists may also help stabilize vulnerable plaques by promoting Calcium transport into cells. This action plays a pivotal role in relieving tension in the tiny vascular smooth muscle, releasing coronary artery spasms, reducing contractions, which increases arterial diameter.

12

Preventable heart attack

But when he sobered up the next morning, Abigail told him everything that had happened. Nabal had a heart attack, and he lay in bed as still as a stone. 1 Samuel, Verse 25:37.

Every day, 100,000 people worldwide experience heart attacks. According to the World Health Organization, 80% of these incidents can be prevented. Just think, if these people had taken the right preventive measures and procedures, 80,000 lives could be saved daily.

Be proactive and take steps to prevent it under any circumstances. If a vulnerable plaque is present, becomes hot and reactive, and experiences additional spasms, it is responsible to take inspired action to address it. If the situation is left unchecked, the heart muscle cells may begin to enter an irreversible scenario due to insufficient blood and oxygen supply.

Imagine a situation where you didn't do your daily respiratory training because of unexpected stress. You started to feel Angina pectoris caused by a spasm of your coronary artery, and you didn't have enough time to reflect on your situation. Maybe you forgot to take your daily medication and supplements, and the increasing distress put you in a harmful spiral. Possibly, you also left your best friend, the Nitroglycerin spray, in your pocket and did not use it to terminate the spasm of your coronary artery and the Angina pectoris chest pain.

Without improvement in oxygen supply, the decrease of blood supply to the part of your heart muscle will progress, and chest pain known as Angina pectoris will worsen.

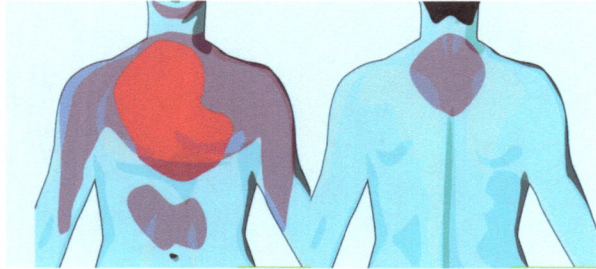

Picture 23. Acute myocardial infarction pain. Front and back of the body, by Hariadhi, Wikimedia.

If you experience symptoms of Angina pectoris, such as chest pain, pressure under your breast-bone, or tightness, and it persists even after using Nitroglycerin spray, taking soluble aspirin, and practicing conscious abdominal breathing, be alert and vigilant. If you do not feel relief within five minutes, it is time to call an ambulance or seek help from your GP or a specialist Cardiologist.

Acting quickly is crucial to protect the heart muscle and prevent damage. If the situation is not addressed promptly and you remain inactive, it can lead to a heart attack, potentially harming your heart muscle.

The image depicts the remaining vitality areas and the possible potential harm in a heart attack.

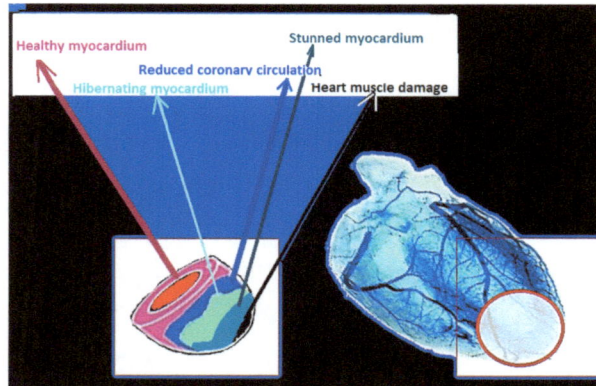

Picture 24. Heart attack viable zones.

The red-rose color represents normal heart tissue with a regular blood supply. The black zone indicates the potentially irreversibly changed part of the heart, where the tissue is dying, and the cells' survival ability is up to six hours. This time frame is crucial for a cardiologist's emergency intervention. The grey-blue zone consists of stunned heart muscle cells with a survival ability of about 72 hours. These cells are shocked and stunned due to the presence of neighboring heart cells that are on the edge of life and death. The turquoise color indicates the surrounding zone of hibernation. The dark blue represents reduced coronary circulation (ischemia), poor blood supply, and low oxygen levels. Under ischemic conditions, the affected cells can stay alive for a few hours longer and, sometimes, even a day or two.

13

Tony's case study

Heal me, LORD, and I will be healed; save me and I will be saved, for you are the one I praise. Jeremiah Chapter17, Verse14.

Tony has for several years not a really healthy lifestyle, a love for food, and sometimes alcohol excess. His lipid levels were elevated, and Tony had a low level of physical exercise. He suffered from time to time episodes of Angina pectoris with low-intensity pain.

Tony also has degenerative changes in both hips and has started to limp. His hip arthritis prevented Tony from exercising and caused a lot of pain even when walking. He was diagnosed with wear and tear hip joints related to aging, and his hip arthritis worsened over time. Tony was also diagnosed with high blood pressure and needed medication, which was insufficient to keep it under control. Tony's blood sugar was elevated, too, and sometimes his GP spoke about borderline Diabetes mellitus.

Two years ago, after he lost his Mum and 3 months later, his Dad has died too. Tony had extreme distress in his family life. The Angina pectoris came then more often and lasted longer; after suffering an intense Angina pectoris episode for more than one hour. Tony was admitted to the hospital and, after that, was referred by his GP for diagnostics, including a non-invasive CT coronary angiography with Calcium score.

He was offered bypass surgery, but at this time, he was not convinced that he needed it. He heard some bad news from his colleagues and friends. They complained about serious complications, including stroke, after undergoing invasive procedures such as balloon angioplasty or bypass surgery.

Tony's report revealed several mixed plaques in his coronary arteries and a high calcium score. The narrowed arteries have a 50 to 70% reduction in diameter, but there was no blockage. Tony's plaques were soft and calcified, and the blood examination showed his body's inflammatory response to this situation.

Tony decided to change his lifestyle. He started to walk more often, but he was limited by hip degenerative disease, so he could not perform full program offered him in form of Cardio exercises. Tony took only occasionally prescribed medication, and he decided to take a full natural medical approach.

Tony changed his diet, and consumed a lot of freshly pressed juices. He purchased several books and self-educated himself about the natural approach to plaques and narrowings of his coronary arteries. It resulted in a reduction of chest pain and body weight.

Then Tony went on holiday to Vietnam and fully immersed himself in the Asian culture, enjoying the delicious food. One evening, after a satisfying meal and a couple of beers, Tony experienced a severe episode of Angina pectoris. He was rushed to a hospital, where he underwent invasive coronary angiography and was offered balloon angioplasty with a balloon-tipped catheter and stent implantation in Vietnam. Tony was initially worried when he was advised against taking a mid-range flight due to the risk. However, after a late-night call to his doctor, who reviewed the coronary angiography report and gave him the green light to fly back home to Australia, Tony realized the seriousness of his Cardio situation. Despite this, he decided not to proceed with the offered procedure and returned home safely.

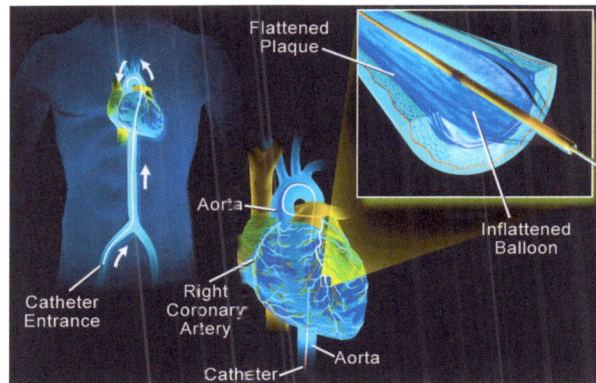

**Picture 25. Balloon tipped catheter. Reverse color view.
By Bruce Blaus. Wikimedia.**

About two months ago, Tony suffered a setback as he suffered another severe Angina pectoris after rich food and clubbing. He took Aspirin and Nitroglycerin spray and phoned the ambulance directly. Tony was treated with Nitroglycerin and oxygen and brought to the hospital. After assessment and triage, he was admitted to the hospital. In the hospital, the doctors observed a slightly elevated troponin marker for diagnosing a heart attack and increased parameters indicating inflammation in his blood.

Tony was treated for a threatening heart attack and spent several days in the hospital, and another invasive coronary angiography was performed. The images showed the same status of coronary arteries with no blockages. Because the blood pressure was volatile, the blood pressure medication was increased, and an additional blood thinner was added to his medication. The doctors and the specialist Cardiologist offered Tony the bypass surgery, but he has not accepted it.

Tony chose to pursue a holistic approach to managing his health instead of opting for bypass surgery. He diligently took his medication and adopted a Cardio diet, which involved reducing his intake of proteins and carbs. Additionally, he sought acupuncture treatment for stress reduction and for hip pain. Additionally, Tony also practiced stress reduction techniques like meditation.

Tony also used Nitroglycerin spray to manage even light episodes of Angina pectoris. To improve his overall fitness, he started walking and engaged in intense respiratory muscle training using oxygen-enriched air from an oxygen concentrator. Furthermore, he began using the treadmill he had purchased a year ago but never used. Tony is committed to his new comprehensive, holistic treatment plan and is dedicated to making lasting changes in his lifestyle.

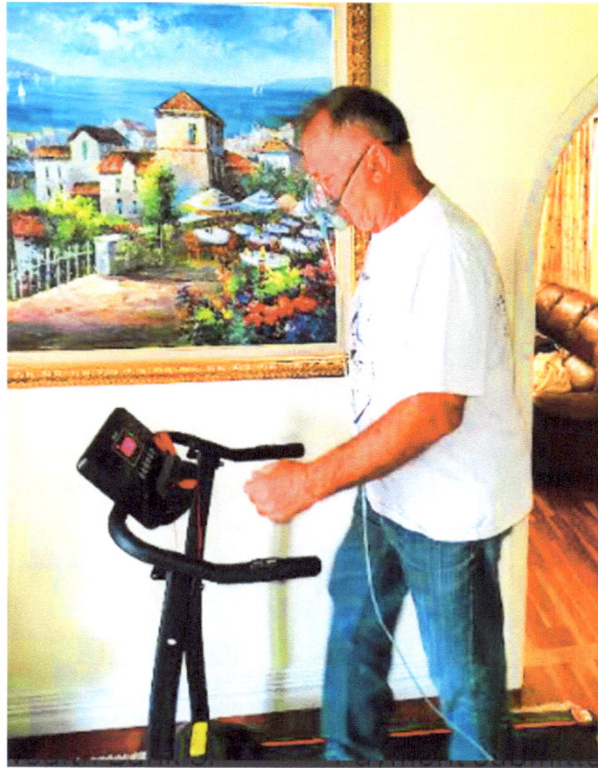

Picture 26. Tony trains on his treadmill. Courtesy Tony.

As a result, Tony can walk better, lose about 8kg of his weight, and decrease the pain in his hip joint by 50 percent. In his new lifestyle, he has no resting Angina pectoris, and he trains on his treadmill every day. Tony's mood has changed, and he is more often happy with his new life. These positive changes in Tony's life are a testimony to the power of lifestyle changes in managing heart conditions.

This is the successful story of how Tone prevented an imminent heart attack and established a new holistic Cardio lifestyle.

14

Your heart positive remodeling

I prayed to you, LORD God, and you healed me. Psalm 30, Verse 2.

Positive remodeling involves restoring your heart to its original healthy condition before adverse remodeling has occurred. This means your next steps will remodel its enlarged shape, soften its hardened structure, restore its natural geometry, and regain your heart's once-missing metabolic flexibility.

You are better now, possible you have taken a significant step by stabilizing the vulnerable plaque and potentially preventing a heart attack threat. You are now in a position of strength, with the confidence that your intelligent heart and your body have the potential to heal and regenerate. You are the knowledgeable observer of your health, empowered to navigate the health care system.

Please remember that the primary aim of positive remodeling is to improve the oxygen supply to your hibernating heart and activate the dormant brain.

Daily respiratory muscle exercises are unparalleled in promoting the positive remodeling of your heart. This includes focusing on abdominal and diaphragmatic breathing. With each breath, essential energy travels through the brain's energy channel known as the microcosmic orbit. It originates from the lower and middle abdomen in the solar plexus, then moves to the groin, ascends along the spine to reach the base of the skull, referred to as the "door to the brain" and finally rises to the highest point of the head before ending at the entry point between the nose and upper lip.

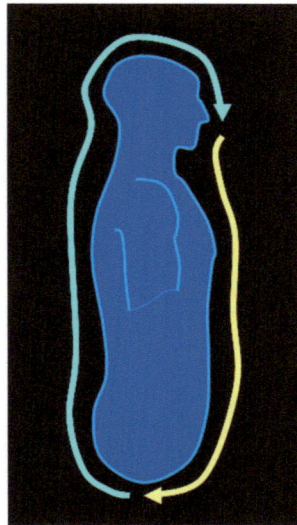

Picture 27. Microcosmic orbit. By Bostjan46. Wikipedia.

During exhalation, the vital energy in the brain channel, a key player in the energy flow, moves down from the bottom lip to the groin and the lower abdomen around the pelvic plexus. If you exhale enough long, up to seven seconds, the energy returns to the top of the head along the spine. The lips, mouth, and tongue connect the front of your body, known as the conception channel, and the back part of your body, the brain energy channel, referred to in traditional medicine as the governing channel, to a perfect functioning microcosmic orbit. This represents the typical flow of vital energy in your microcosmic orbit. Visualizing this continuous flow can effectively energize your body.

There is no better time than now to prioritize your heart health by starting an exercise routine. This step marks your entry into a 21st-century, holistic treatment plan and sets the stage for your heart's positive remodeling.

It is indisputable that regular, appropriate exercise is essential for heart health. But, whatever fitness system you choose, you will always benefit from breathing correctly during your routine.

During exercise, focus your awareness on bodily functions and practice abdominal breathing. Apply abdominal breathing during walking, energy channel training, interval training, yoga, and

Pilates. Be aware of the value of respiratory muscle training during yoga, active meditation, or any other physical activity.

Correct breathing can activate your body's immune system, prevent viral or bacterial infections, and reduce stress. It can also strengthen your connection with the fabric of the Universe and support its healing powers.

In addition to your daily practice of abdominal and orbital breathing, the best way to start your training is with a gentle set of exercises that improve your spine flexibility, increase the range of motion in your shoulders, and enhance the function of your heart. The description of the spine flow moves (SFM) will follow in the next chapter.

15

Training for your intelligent heart

For physical training is of some value, but godliness (spiritual training) is of value in everything and in every way, since it holds promise for the present life and for the life to come. 1 Timothy Chapter 4, Verse 8.

This is an introduction to Spine Flow Moves (SFM). The technique was first introduced to the author of this book by Dr. Sushil Bhutacharaya, a renowned yoga teacher. Over time and through the author's increasing experiences, it has been modified to ensure safe performance for those with adverse heart remodeling and other heart-related issues.

Spine flow moves consists of circular and coordinated exercises that target all sections of the spine, improving flexibility and heart function. It is important to gradually increase the number of movements each week or every two weeks. Patience and dedication are crucial during this process, as it signifies your progress in strength and flexibility, ultimately leading to improved heart health. It is essential that you perform these exercises only to the extent that feels comfortable and without any exertion. This is vital to prevent any strain and discomfort, and to ensure a safe and beneficial practice for your heart health.

Tracing circles with the hips

Stand with your feet wide apart and point your toes straight ahead. Place your hands on your hips. Move your hips in a big circle several times, first clockwise and then counter clockwise.

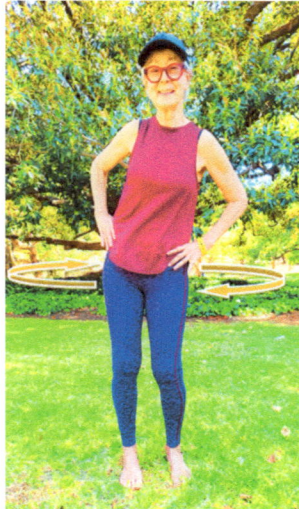

Picture 28. Elly circles her hips.

Tracing circles with the knees.

Place your feet side by side, almost together, and keep your knees together. Bend your knees slightly (soft knees) and clasp them with your thumbs on the inside. It is essential to keep your upper body slightly bent, with your head erect as far as possible, your neck relaxed, and your eyes fixed on any point at the height of your head. Please do not look down on your feet. Please stay relax with the core of your body while you maintain control and focus during the exercise.

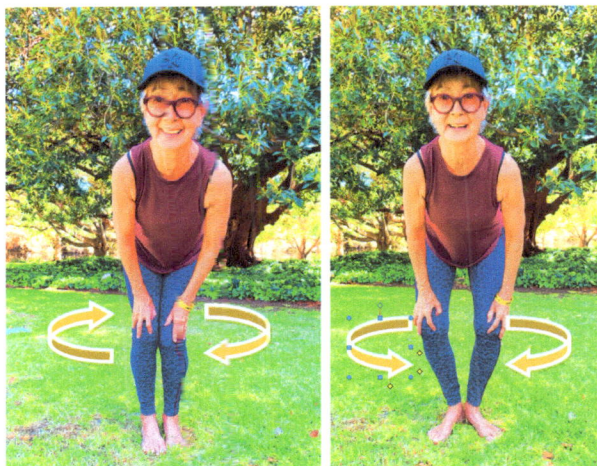

Picture 29. Elly circles with her knees.

Move your knees held together in a circle several times clockwise, then repeat the exercise in the opposite direction. Remember to breathe abdominal during the workout. Then, move your feet out to create an angle of 80 degrees. Keep your heels together, and turn your soft knees with your thumbs on the inside of both knees. Keep the upper body straight and still during this movement, with the head erect as far as possible, neck relaxed, and eyes gently fixed on a point straight ahead.

Move your knee inwards, tracing a circle clockwise several times, and then repeat it in the opposite direction by tracing circles outwards with your knees. During this exercise, keep doing your abdominal breathing.

Keep your head still. Gradually and gently increase the speed of your hip movements while staying coordinated. The movement should come from the energy center of your body, which includes the solar plexus and pelvic plexus inside your belly, a few centimeters below, above, and around your belly button.

Tracing circles with your shoulder.

Stand with your feet wide apart and point your toes straight ahead. Hang your hands alongside your hips. Move your left shoulder in a circle several times, first clockwise and then counter clockwise. Repeat it please with your right shoulder.

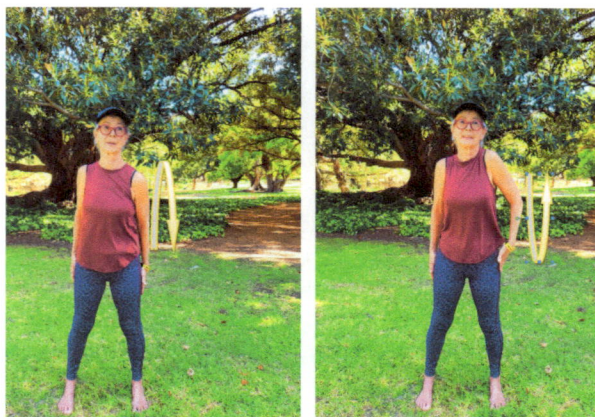

Picture 30. Elly circles her shoulder.

Tracing circles with your arms up, locked as close as possible to the head.

With the feet wider apart, toes pointing straight ahead, lift arms. Lock thumbs together, arms straight above the head touching your ears. Begin moving sideways to the right, bending from the waist as far as you can, then extend the bend, twisting from the hips down to the right. Please do a circle moving to the left only as far as you can go, then begin to straighten without tipping backward and complete the circle. During this exercise, the arms are kept straight and as close as possible the ears. Breathe in when upright and out when bent. Repeat the exercise in an anticlockwise direction.

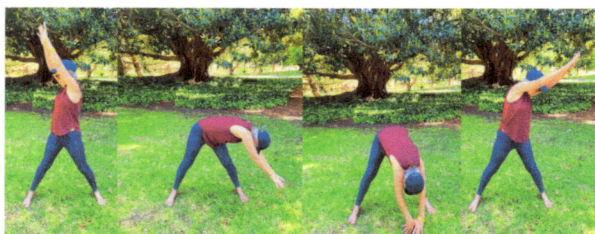

Picture 31. Elly tracing her arms locked to the head.

Tracing circles with your elbows.

With feet shoulder-width apart, toes pointing straight ahead, lift arms, elbows bent, fingers on the shoulders. Keep your eyes open during the exercise—stay fully aware. Bring elbows together while the chin moves toward the chest. As you move the elbows up, try to look through the triangle created by the elbows. Open the elbows and circle outwards, stretching the shoulders. Repeat the exercise by tracing circles outwards. This exercise benefits your heart in an extraordinary way.

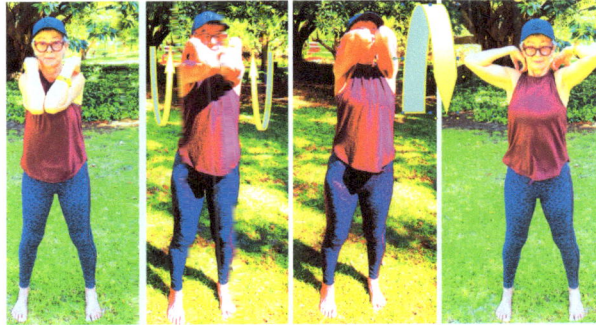

Picture 22. Eily circles with her elbows.

Kissing shoulders.

These are easy moves that are also fun. Lift arms with bent elbows and down-facing hands up to the chest until hands meet in the middle. For the exercise, separate hands, keeping arms parallel, by moving elbows back as far as possible to allow the shoulder blades to 'kiss.' Breathe in and lift the chest when arms open and out when hands come together. Repeat it several times. The kissing shoulder moves bring warmth to the shoulders and relieve heart, shoulders, and chest problems, all while being an enjoyable activity.

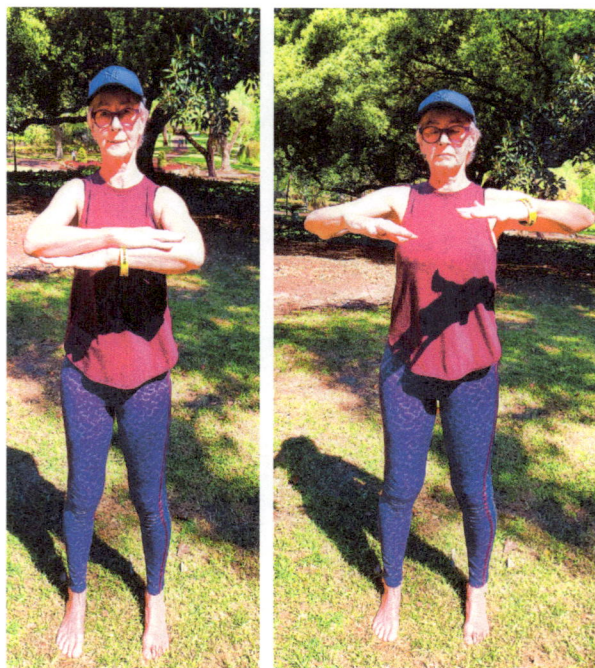

Picture 33. Elly does make kissing shoulders.

Head rolls.

Remember the following instructions for the head roll exercise: exercise caution and start with gentle, tiny circles. To minimize the risk of being lightheaded, perform these exercises at the beginning while sitting. Stand with your feet shoulder-width apart, toes pointing straight ahead, and fold your arms across your chest with your shoulders relaxed. Move your head sideways towards the right shoulder, bringing it as close as possible to the shoulder without lifting it.

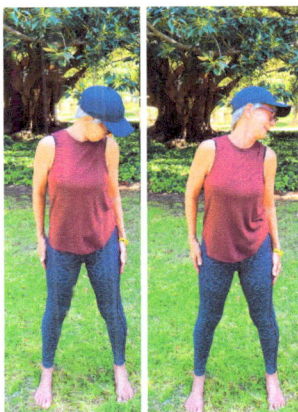

**Picture 34. Elly does make
the head rolls.**

Then, trace a circle across the chest and up the left side. Repeat the moves several times. Keep your eyes gently fixed on a horizontal point straight ahead. These neck and head movements benefit all ear problems, improve the blood supply to the brain, and boost communication between the heart and brain.

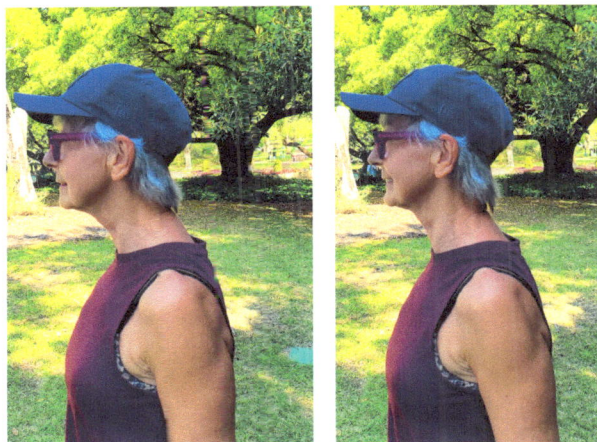

Picture 35. Elly performs a turtle move of her neck.

Turtle moves.

Then, in the end, move your head forward and stretch your neck out as far as possible forward, like a turtle, several times.

PLEASE NOTE that you should perform all exercises only to extend as far as possible and effortlessly to avoid any stress and pain.

16

Acupuncture for stress

Do not be anxious about anything. Instead, in every situation, through prayer and petition with thanksgiving, tell your requests to God . Philippians Chapter 4, Verse 6.

Medical acupuncture is a therapeutic procedure that uses the energy channels of your body and its specific points to regulate bodily functions. Your energy channels are connected to major sensory and motor nerves, which act as pathways for vital energy flow. According to 21st-century medical research, they are connected to your brain, heart, and spinal cord. The solar plexus in the belly and the pelvic plexus below the navel are also specialized neuronal centers that link your heart, brain, and spine through these energy channels.

During acupuncture, thin, sterile needles are inserted into the entry points to stimulate your body's self-organizing system. These points serve as gateways between your body's internal and external environments. They are equipped with exceptional sensors and a rich network of blood vessels that connect directly to your heart and brain.

Acupuncture intervention can either speed up or slow down the normal functions of body parts or internal organs. Nerves, blood, and bodily fluids like lymphatic fluid, which contains water, minerals, and small molecules such as oxygen (O2) and Nitric Oxide (NO), are responsible for carrying out these functions. Additionally, biochemical mediators and hormones like endorphins are involved. Endorphins help to alleviate pain, reduce stress, and enhance overall well-being. When the body is distressed, an acupuncture needle can help to decrease the intensity of the energy flow. The communication between nerve cells and neurons happens wireless through electromagnetic waves, similar to how antennas transmit signals. Nerve roots transmit impulses to your muscles and internal organs via electrical currents.

Acupuncture plays a pivotal role in regulating your body's energy exchange, thereby maintaining its integrity. The entry points, which are energetic and informational centers, are equipped with unique anatomical structures, abundant sensors and receptors, a rich blood vessel network, and specialized nerves. These points can adjust the flow of vital energy, its intake, and distribution. The communication and the vital energy flow freely alongside your body and concentrate at the entry points to the energy channels. These specific points also have the ability to respond effectively to the needles inserted during acupuncture.

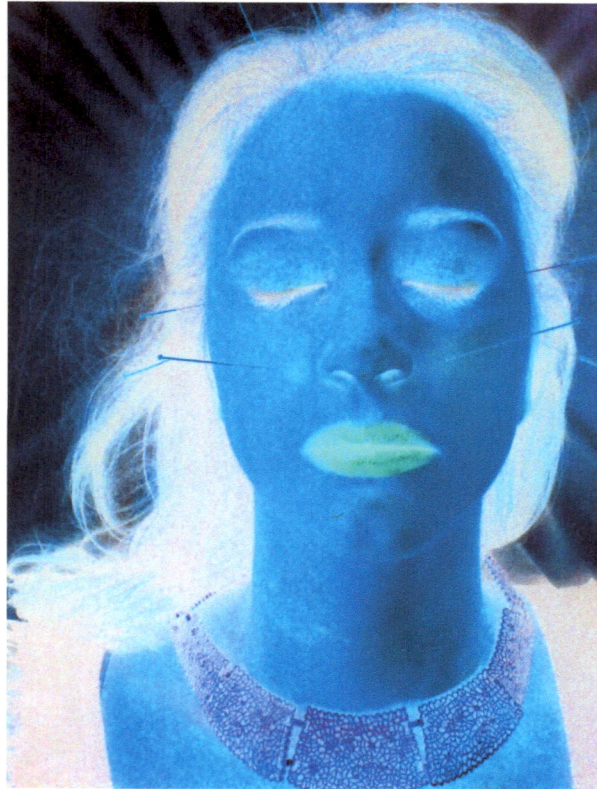

Picture 37. Acupuncture for stress reduction.

The author's book "Grace in movement", published in August 2024, provides more knowledge about your energy channels.

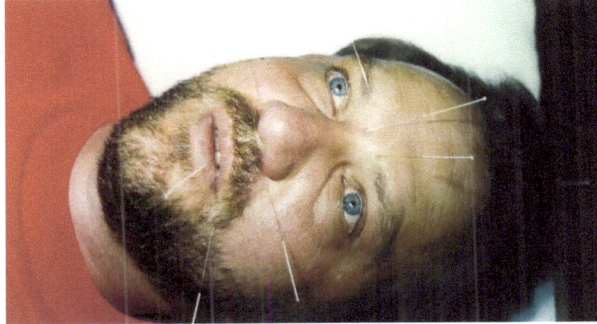

Picture 38. Acupuncture for stress reduction.

17

Your heart's regenerative power

Jesus answered: Very truly I tell you, no one can enter the kingdom of God unless they are born of water and the Spirit. Flesh gives birth to flesh, but the Spirit gives birth to spirit. You should not be surprised at my saying: You must be born again. The wind blows wherever it pleases. You hear its sound, but you cannot tell where it comes from or where it is going. So it is with everyone born of the Spirit. John Chapter 3, Verse 3-8.

Your incredible heart beats tirelessly for over 90 or even 100 years, continually regenerating itself. In 2010, Harvard University made a groundbreaking revelation that every heart produces adult omnipotent stem cells, which play a crucial role in regenerating and restoring damaged heart tissue.

This discovery led to extensive research into stem cells and their regenerative potential for all internal organs. In 2012, the Nobel Prize was awarded to John B. Gurdon and Dr Shinya Yamanaka for their work in reprogramming ordinary cells into stem cells that can regenerate all internal organs of the human body.

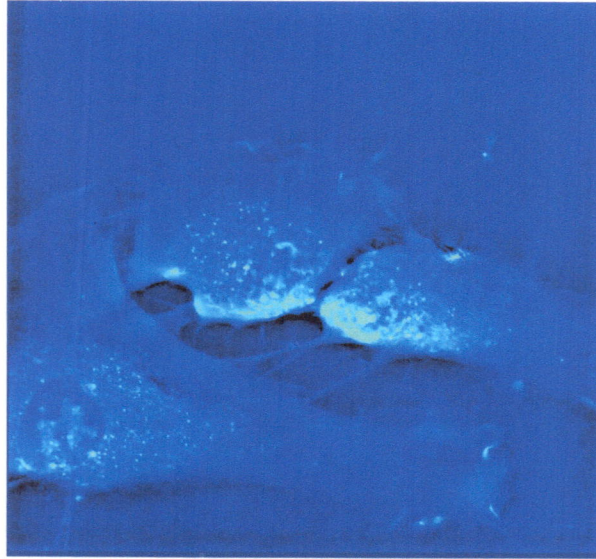

Picture 39. Stem cells. Wikipedia.

Organs like the liver, kidney, and spleen also produce adult omnipotent stem cells, contributing to the body's lifelong renewal capacity. Even slow-regenerating organs, such as the heart and the brain, have the ability to renew and regenerate over time. For example, the heart takes about 20 years for complete renewal, while the brain's regeneration process takes approximately 40 years to exchange all neurons and nerve cells.

This research underscores the remarkable regenerative potential of your body, including the possibility of the brain regenerating multiple times over a long lifetime with a healthy lifestyle.

In Volume 6, page 78 of the book entitled *Life and Teachings of the Masters of the Far East by Baird* Spalding published in 1991 we find a most excellent description of the stem cells.

As the cell divides and creates a new cell, our thought is implanted upon it...In the first cell, all is perfect. That cell was first known as the Christ cell." (i.e. the anointed cell) *"It is always just as young as ever it was. It never takes on old age. It is the primal spark of life. When we implant in it our thoughts of limitation or old age, or any condition outside of perfection, the body responds. Cells born from the first cell take on its image. Originally it is the image and likeness of God. It is perfect in every way. But it becomes the form we carry in our minds...if we carry the image of perfection always, what will it do for these cells? It will build perfection.*

18

Your heart's protective hormones

The heart's hormones play a essential role in the body's hormonal regulation. Every 24 to 48 minutes, the heart produces four hormones that go beyond metabolism and energy production. These hormones influence the stress response, fat metabolism, blood acidity/alkalinity, tissue oxygenation equilibrium, and water/minerals balance.

The heart produces four major independent hormones: atrial natriuretic peptide type A, brain natriuretic peptide type B (BNP), which was discovered in the brain but actually originates from the heart, type C ,first extracted from salmon, this is why the salmon is healthy for your heart, and type D, a close relative of a hormone found in the green mamba.

Brain Natriuretic Peptide (BNP) helps the body compensate for heart weakness. Blood BNP measurements aid doctors in diagnosing and treating various heart conditions. Heart weakness occurs when the heart becomes too lazy or stiff due to hibernating myocardium, preventing it from pumping normally. The most common causes for increased blood BNP are coronary artery disease and high blood pressure (hypertension).

The additional fifth hormone produced by the heart accelerates the production of adenosine triphosphate (ATP) to fuel cellular breathing. Increased oxygen intake enhances the production of high-energy ATP available for all cells in the body.

In emergencies, the heart can produce two additional hormones, cardiomyosin and serum response factor, to protect itself. These hormones act as protectors, limiting the blood supply to the brain when it becomes selfish and demands excessive blood and energy at the expense of the heart and other internal organs.

19

Your heart's spiritual healing

The light of the body is the eye: therefore when your eye is single, your whole body also is full of light; but when your eye is evil, your body also is full of darkness. Luke Chapter 11, Verse 34.

Spirituality is not just a feeling or belief in something beyond 3 dimensional space and time. It is a profound recognition that it can transform your life. It is the divine WHOLE, transcending your individual existence.

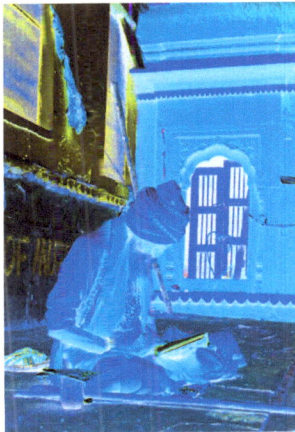

Picture 40. People of Varanasi. Wikipedia.

Embracing spirituality opens the door for you to a deeper understanding of your life and the fabric of the Universe. The shift to a world beyond three dimensions can occur during experiences such as falling in love, deep compassion for others, meditation or prayer, medical acupuncture, energy channel training, or intense respiratory muscle training (orbital breathing).

It is important to remember that your breathing technique is not just a physical act, but a gateway to spiritual development. The discovery of orbital breathing, a method where you sense and visualize your breath moving in a circular path alongside your bodily micro-orbit, is a life-changing experience. Expertise in orbital breathing can give you the experience of an energy shower, a burst of energy all over your body, starting from your head and shoulders and descending to your toes.

As you nurture your awareness of your body's interior, you will come to understand the deep connection between your heart, brain, and spirituality. With the evolution of your spiritual practice, you will be able to feel the life force pulsating through your revitalized body. This can lead you to an integrative quantum experience, a new dimension in your body's sensation. Once you reach this state of joy, you will be in a position to recreate this experience. These bio-energetic experiences for your body will be a constant source of joy during your spine flow moves, orbital breathing and spiritual training.

Spiritual and mental strength training are important parts of reversing adverse remodeling of your heart. First, staying grounded in your intelligent heart and acting as an impartial observer is essential. When your mind, heart and spirit are in a neutral observer position, your body will be more in harmony. When you repeat this attitude more times, it will create a sense of well-being and better health.

Remember, the WHOLE is greater than the sum of its parts.

Both modern science and ancient wisdom agree that disconnecting from your 3-D space-time conditioned mindset allows your heart to connect with the fabric of the Universe, leading to a dimension of perfect harmony.

Be aware that you can transform the power of negativity into your personal growth. Bridging the gap between your mind and heart is vital for spiritual healing.

Achieving unity between your body, heart, mind, spirit, and soul is a profound accomplishment. Your ability to overcome adverse heart remodeling also relies on your spiritual skills, intelligence, and resilience against external influences.

Surround yourself with supportive individuals whose collective wisdom will help your healing process, empowering you to triumph over the factors that led to adverse heart remodeling.

Understanding 'individual oneness' and its role in healing is essential. It allows you to embrace your unique qualities and align your actions and intentions with your heart. Simplifying the meaning of healing your mind from "optionality," it is good to be genuine, maintain a consistent personality, and avoid having conflicting attitudes in your behavior.

By referencing the Bible's teachings about health and the body, we can better understand individual oneness and see things in a simple, single-minded way.

The best example of the spiritual healing and transformation is Elly's dream from early September 2024. Elly's case study and her spiritual development was described in the Chapter 7.

I walked down to a unit that should be my home. It was dark, sad, heavy, and ugly. I felt I deserved it, what else? I continued exploring my home and found my garden, but it looked dead.

Then something strange happened, and I saw through my eyes that everything was full of light and had turned into beautiful art. It was a breathtaking, magnificent moment. It was huge. I looked and looked, and it became even more beautiful. I was in awe and felt wonder and joy.

My attention turned to a basin with running tap water. It was just pouring out. Seeing the water running, I panicked, only to find a plug shaped like Jesus in a robe. This plug looked like beautiful artwork, too. I felt it was bad to use such a plug of great significance. After a few moments of hesitating, I cautiously placed the plug in the basin, and the water stopped running. I was relieved. And then I saw that my new garden was alive and beautiful. My suburb also changed to a lovely, healthy environment, and I was safe. I became proud to see all these wonderful changes.

About the author

Dr. Jerzy (George) Dyczynski, MD, MBA, is a highly experienced medical doctor with a deep interest and extensive experience in conventional and traditional medical practices. He began his career as a medical doctor in 1976, became a specialist in internal medicine in 1987, and became a Cardiologist in 2002. Dr Jerzy has worked in healthcare settings in Poland, Germany, Switzerland, and Australia, refining his skills and knowledge. Dr. Jerzy holds a Doctorate in Cardiology, has authored numerous papers in international journals, and has delivered many scientific presentations. He has also received qualifications in medical quality management from the Bavarian Medical Council in Munich and earned a medical MBA from the University of Lueneburg in Germany. Dr. Jerzy Dyczynski has worked for over 35 years as a Medical Doctor, Specialist in Internal Medicine, and Cardiologist in public and private healthcare systems. He also researched Heart-Brain Medicine and worked as a clinical acupuncturist at the ECU clinic for outpatients at Edith Cowan University in Perth between 2008 and 2009. His extensive training in traditional Chinese medicine, energy channels, traditional gymnastics for health, and Kung Fu martial arts over 30 years has provided him with a unique perspective on holistic health, which he integrates into his cardiology practice to provide comprehensive care for his patients. He is also an author, having published several books integrating Eastern and Western medicine. His most recent books include "The Dyczynski Program: Healing the Intelligent Heart", published in 2022, and the following book, "Grace in Movement," published in 2024, which focuses on the integration of traditional and conventional modern medicine.

www.ingramcontent.com/pod-product-compliance
Lightning Source LLC
Chambersburg PA
CBHW061136030426
42334CB00003B/60